YOUR KNOWLEDGE HAS VALUE

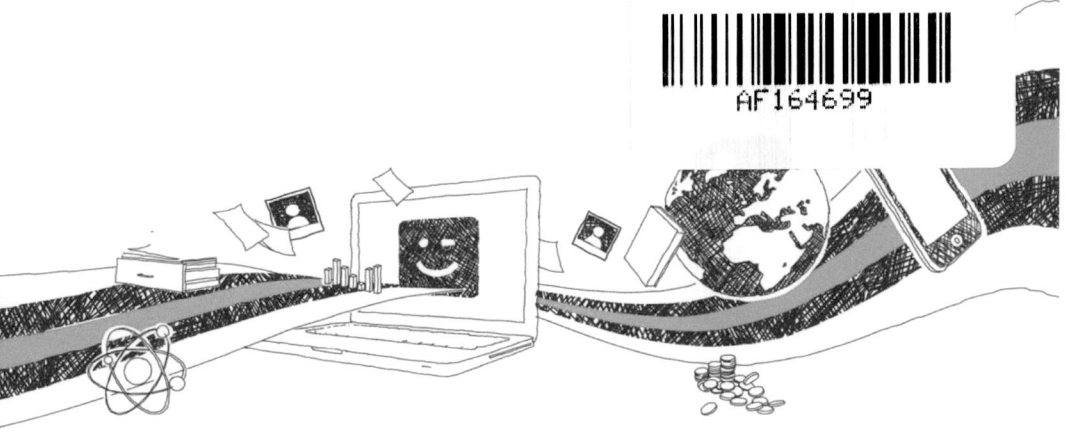

- We will publish your bachelor's and master's thesis, essays and papers

- Your own eBook and book - sold worldwide in all relevant shops

- Earn money with each sale

Upload your text at www.GRIN.com
and publish for free

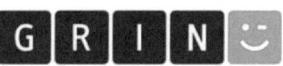

Bibliographic information published by the German National Library:

The German National Library lists this publication in the National Bibliography; detailed bibliographic data are available on the Internet at http://dnb.dnb.de .

This book is copyright material and must not be copied, reproduced, transferred, distributed, leased, licensed or publicly performed or used in any way except as specifically permitted in writing by the publishers, as allowed under the terms and conditions under which it was purchased or as strictly permitted by applicable copyright law. Any unauthorized distribution or use of this text may be a direct infringement of the author s and publisher s rights and those responsible may be liable in law accordingly.

Imprint:

Copyright © 2017 GRIN Verlag, Open Publishing GmbH
Print and binding: Books on Demand GmbH, Norderstedt Germany
ISBN: 9783668585232

This book at GRIN:

http://www.grin.com/en/e-book/381238/the-evidence-for-the-safety-and-efficacy-of-metal-on-metal-hip-prostheses

Patrick Kimuyu

The Evidence for the Safety and Efficacy of Metal-On-Metal Hip Prostheses

GRIN Publishing

GRIN - Your knowledge has value

Since its foundation in 1998, GRIN has specialized in publishing academic texts by students, college teachers and other academics as e-book and printed book. The website www.grin.com is an ideal platform for presenting term papers, final papers, scientific essays, dissertations and specialist books.

Visit us on the internet:

http://www.grin.com/

http://www.facebook.com/grincom

http://www.twitter.com/grin_com

Evidence for the Safety and Efficacy of Metal-On-Metal Hip Prostheses: Sufficient or Insufficient?

Name: Patrick K. Kimuyu

Inhaltsverzeichnis

Abstract 3

Introduction 4

Materials and Design 4

Clinical Safety and Efficacy 5

Conclusion 10

References 11

Abstract
Introduction

Metal-on-metal prostheses have been in use since 1960's, and their safety and efficacy has never been reviewed adequately. The current reports of metal-on-metal hip implants' failure have led to health concerns

Materials and Design

Materials used in the analysis were the Cormet Hip Resurfacing System and Birmingham Hip Resurfacing System. Literature materials were analyzed using the Cox regression model.

Critical Safety and Efficacy

Literature sources indicate that, the failures observed in the two metal-on-metal hip devices can be attributed to the lack of efficient regulatory policies. Epidemiological reports indicate that most patients around the globe have experienced the adverse effects of metal-on-metal hip implants.

It is argued that, FDA failed to carry out comprehensive evaluation on the safety and efficacy of metal-on-metal hip devices before their approval to reduce the health risks associated to the devices.

Evidence to the insufficiency of the evidence provided by the regulatory agencies can be provided by the confession of the duPuy's designer. Recently, he admitted that the devices should not be in use today because they encompass enormous defaults.

Conclusion

The procedure of technology assessment has been found to have been based on inappropriate scientific evidence. Cormet 2000 and the BHR devices' technology assessment did not meet all the required criteria. Therefore, evidence for the safety and efficacy of metal-on-metal hip prostheses in 2005 was insufficient.

Introduction

Metal-on-metal hip prostheses have been in use clinical since 1960s, and its literature review has been showing diverse changes. Clinical studies have been conducted to ascertain the usefulness of the technology in regard to its safety and efficacy (Amstutz & LeDuff 2006). Ordinarily, metal-on-metal total hip implants are believed to release toxic substances in the patient's body, causing significant health concerns of the technology. Cohen (2012, par. 1) reaffirms "thousands of patients around the world may have been exposed to toxic substances after being implanted with poorly regulated and potentially dangerous hip devices." Therefore, this paper will provide a critical review on the evidence for the safety and efficacy of metal-on-metal hip prostheses, primarily with regard to its insufficiency.

Materials and Design

Analysis of the literature involved the use of different literature sources, which were analyzed using the Cox regression model.

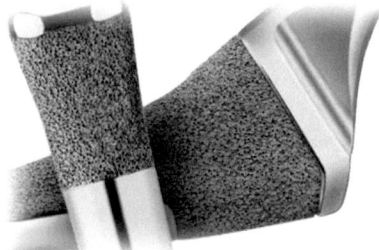

Figure 1: Trabecular Metal™ Primary Hip Prosthesis

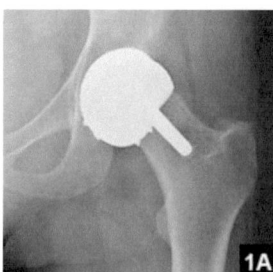

Figure 2: Cormet 2000 device on the femoral cup (Allan et al. 2009)

Device Composition

Metal-on-metal Hip Device	Device Composition
Cormet Hip Resurfacing System	Metal femoral and acetabular component
Birmingham Hip Resurfacing System	Metal femoral and acetabular component

Clinical Safety and Efficacy

Literature materials indicate that, FDA has not been able to design efficient regulatory measures aimed at reducing the risk posed by metal-on-metal hip arthroplasty. For instance, reports indicate that FDA was aware of the safety and efficacy issues related to metal-on-metal hip arthroplasty, but it maintained that there was a need for scientific data to unravel the mystery surrounding the technology. Surprisingly, FDA seems to have neglected the issue and continued to allow clearance of metal-on-metal hip implants for marketing. It is argued that FDA carries the blame for the damage incurred over the last thirty years for failing in its primary mission. In this case, the agency did not apply ethical standards in allowing clearance for metal-on-metal hip implants. It is argued that they were "fully aware of the deadly risks in use of toxic metal device failures for these implants, but the agency failed in its primary mission and continued to allow massive proliferation with full FDA clearance for marketing, unfettered by oversight" (Schrag 2013, p. 2).

Recently, Thomas P. Schmalzried astonished the public and healthcare professionals by testifying in the Chicago's court case that he "had to revise 15 out of 66 insertions (23 percent failure rate), which he said, is an unacceptable failure rate" (Schrag 2013, p. 3). Ironically, FDA provided full market clearance for metal-on-metal hip implants in 2005, leading to the release of over 34,000 metal-on-metal devices in the United States. Schrag (2013, p. 3) reports "in a separate news report dated April 2, 2013, Dr. Schmalzried further testified that he would not use ASR and that its benefits do not outweigh the risk." This testimony provides evidence to the safety and efficacy concerns on the metal-on-metal hip implants, but FDA seems to have neglected the risks associated with the implants for total hip replacement (Duncan et al. 2010).

Ideally, FDA based its evidence on the benefits of metal-on-metal hip implants for total hip replacement. Currently, metal-on-metal hip implants are used as a reliable alternative for total hip replacement (Bruening et al. 2006). Despite the failure rates observed by surgeons in 1980s, total hip replacement prostheses gained popularity in 1990s because of their usefulness in treating young and active patients (Dettori et al. 2013).

From a clinical perspective, the use of total hip replacement, primarily metal-on-metal hip devices has several advantages compared to the hip resurfacing (Bozic et al. 2010). For instance, it has been reported that metal-on-metal hip implants "provide the ability to use large diameter femoral head sizes compared to other articulating combinations" (Dettori et al. p. 21). In addition, metal-on-metal hip implants have large sizes, which are believed to mimic the patient's natural anatomy. Therefore, they reduce post-operative dislocation through the improvement of the joint stability (Lee, McIsaac & Noseworthy 2007).

Despite the benefits associated with metal-on-metal hip implants, they encompass enormous safety concerns because they produce metal ions such as Chromium and Cobalt, which cause peri-prosthetic tissue and bone destruction (Brazzelli et al. 2004). Therefore, evidence for the safety and efficacy of metal-on-metal hip prostheses released in 2005 appears to be insufficient in various perspectives.

Insufficiency of the evidence for the safety and efficacy of metal-on-metal hip prostheses can be explained by highlighting on the safety concerns associated with the procedures. It is suggested that FDA should have followed Technology Assessment guidelines before the approval of metal-on-metal hip implants for commercial production. In addition, it should have evaluated the devices design, uncertain risks from metal ions and post-marketing surveillance to reduce its safety risks on patients.

It is argued that regulators in the United States and Europe did not identify the tweaked designs by manufacturers of metal-on-metal hip implants before granting them approval, and yet the designers were aware of the dangers. These design changes are believed to have encompassed enormous consequences on the patients' safety. Cohen (2012, par. 27) reports "instead of alerting regulators and patients to their concerns, companies tweaked the design of their total hip implants." One surgeon who had been using metal-on-metal hip implants was quoted saying, "We are seeing patients with tapers which are blackened, destroyed, metal getting into the tissues of the hip, damaging the muscles, taking out some of the bone, so destroying parts of the pelvis" (Cohen 2012, par. 32). Research studies indicate that, Cobalt and Chromium ions are carcinogenic because they were found to cause genotoxic changes in animals (Dayan & Paine 2001). However, regulatory agencies in the United Kingdom noticed that fact recently after the

London Implant Retrieval Centre confirmed the release of trivalent Chromium ions by the metal-on-metal hip implants (Ladon et al 2004). Therefore, the high failure rate of metal-on-metal hip implants was attributable to the release of the genotoxic metal ions during the post-operative period (Amstutz, Ball & LeDuff 2007).

According to dePuy's designer Dr. Schmalzried, Cobalt release by the device is relatively low, primarily in patients whose devices function well. He states that patients with well-functioning metal-to-metal hip implants do not record his level of Cobalt ions in their blood circulations (Antoniou et al. 2008). However, "studies show that blood Cobalt concentrations generated through the wear of some of the newer metal-on-metal total hip prostheses can reach over 300µg/L, higher than anything routinely documented in the past" (Cohen 2012, par. 21). Surprisingly, regulatory agencies in Europe and the U.S failed to identify the genotoxic aspect of the metal-on-metal hip implants before approval in 2005, leading the current health consequences.

On the other hand, the criteria used in assessing the safety and efficacy of metal-on-metal hip prostheses in 2005 were not sufficient. It has been found that, the approved prostheses met only one of the five criteria used in determining the safety and efficacy of new technologies applied in for hip arthroplasty.

According to the California Technology Assessment Forum, the Birmingham Hip Resurfacing (BHR) and Cormet 2000 devices met the first technology assessment criterion, which requires government regulatory bodies to approve new technologies used for prosthetic purposes before allowing manufacturers to produce them for marketing. On 9 May, 2006, the Birmingham Hip Resurfacing System received FDA's pre-market approval although there were several conditions (Back et al. 2005). Some of these conditions included the implementation of a training program to provide a comprehensive analysis of the adverse effects. In addition, a learning curve was to be evaluated to determine the safety and efficacy of the technology (Karliner 2010).

On the other hand, the Cormet Hip Resurfacing (Cormet 2000) System was approved on 3 July, 2007 after a comprehensive review of two post-approval studies. In addition to the two post-approval studies, FDA required the Cormet 2000 producer and other healthcare stakeholders to establish strategies for performance assessment, primarily under the appropriate conditions (CTAF 2007).

However, the technology assessment of the Birmingham Hip Resurfacing and the Cormet Hip Resurfacing systems did not meet the other four TA criteria. For instance, Technology Assessment criterion 2, which requires the approval of prosthetic technologies to be based on scientific evidence regarding health outcome, was not met. Ordinarily, scientific evidence serves a significant role in designing technologies used in healthcare for treatment of different health conditions (Back, Bare & Shimmin 2005). As such, conclusions on the safety and efficacy of the new technology's approval are based on sufficient scientific evidence.

From a scientific perspective, the approval of Cormet 2000 and BHR devices was not based on valid scientific evidence because there were no randomized trials conducted to evaluate their safety. It was based on few case studies. In addition, these case studies have been identified to have been conducted by a single surgeon contrary to the requirements of technology assessment requirements, which include an array of peer-reviewed literature. The peer-reviewed literature in this case consisted of level-five evidence, which is not considered to be appropriate for comprehensive technology assessment. Instead, level-1 evidence was not included in the peer-reviewed literature, which was used to approve Cormet 2000 and BHR devices. Researchers argue that, evidence for safety and efficacy of hip resurfacing could have been obtained by comparing it with the total hip arthroplasty. It is believed that, the evidence required for generating comprehensive conclusions on the safety and efficacy of the BHR and Cormet 2000 could have been obtained through a multi-site RCT of the technologies compared to the studies involving patients under total hip arthroplasty treatment. The significance of using level-1 studies in technology assessment includes the identification of the technology benefits regarding to the core health outcomes. Secondly, they help in determining whether the new technology holds more benefits than the existing technologies (CTAF 2007).

The second failure associated with the technology assessment of Cormet 2000 and BHR devices was that it did not meet criterion three. In criterion 3, the new technology is investigated to ensure that it provides significant improvement on the net health outcomes. For instance, there were no Randomized Clinical Trials which were published before the FDA approval of the two devices. This is one of the principal factors as to why the metal-on-metal resurfacing procedures were discovered to encompass safety concerns long after their approval for use in total hip replacement (Girard, Lavigne & Venditolli 2006). Moreover, some case-study reports indicate that metal-on-metal resurfacing procedures had proved to be ineffective in case series conducted between 1998 and 2000 (Daniel, McMinn & Pynsent 2004). These reports indicate that 70 percent of the 45 Japanese patients who participated in the trials developed dysplasia while 4 percent were reported to have osteoarthritis without dysplasia. Therefore, California Technology Assessment Forum concludes that, evidenced for safety and efficacy for metal-on-metal hip prostheses is insufficient because it does not address the issue of health outcomes (CTAF 2007).

Moreover, Cormet 2000 and BHR devices did not meet the requirements of TA criterion 4, which requires the new technology to possess equal benefits to the existing alternative technology. It has been reported that metal-on-metal devices approved by FDA have fewer benefits than the old procedure of total hip arthroplasty (Kaulback, Levin & Sehatzadeh 2012). This has been evidenced by the inability of Cormet 2000 and BHR to alleviate hip pain in patients. It is also believed that these technologies record low improvement of the patient's function compared to total hip arthroplasty procedures. Therefore, hip resurfacing is regarded as the most preferable treatment alternative for active patients, as long as they meet all the qualifications required for total hip arthroplasty because revision procedures produce successful treatment outcomes (CTAF 2007).

It has also been argued that the FDA approval of metal-on-metal resurfacing procedures was based on evidence obtained from investigational settings only. Ordinarily, new technologies are expected to improve health outcomes outside of the investigational setting although they may show significant improvement under investigational setting. California Technology Assessment Forum argues that, FDA' approval of metal-on-metal hip resurfacing did not include adequate technology assessment procedures to ensure the aspect of improving health outcomes is met before its release for clinical use (CTAF 2007). This is probably the reason why numerous hip replacement surgeries have failed.

Currently, critics claim that the American and European regulators failed to enforce post-marketing surveillance in providing evidence for the safety and efficacy of metal-on-metal hip prostheses in 2005 when the duPuy device was first released. Cohen (2012, par. 59) reports "the regulators mandated no post-approval studies requiring careful follow-up of patients implanted with devices capable of producing toxic debris." Meanwhile, FDA is seeking for decisions on the classification of hip prostheses. In addition, FDA is designing policies to ensure that hip prostheses are regulated efficiently in the future.

Conclusion

In conclusion, it seems correct that the evidence provided for the safety and efficacy of metal-on-metal hip prostheses in 2005 was insufficient. It has been reported that millions of patients have experienced adverse consequences after the implantation of metal-on-metal hip implants.

Therefore, the insufficiency of the evidence can be attributed to the failure by the regulatory agencies which did not consider all the required procedures before the approval of the devices. It is quite surprising to learn that the designer of the duPuy device admits that the device encompasses numerous faults, which are believed to be the principal cause of the high failure rate.

References

Allan, G, Hulsen, J, Mai, M & Milbrandt, J 2009, Acetabular cup malalignment after total hip resurfacing arthroplasty: a case for elective revision?, *Orthopedics,* vol. 32, no. 11, par. 1-18, viewed 15 October 2017, Healio database, doi: 10.3928/01477447-20090922-22.

Amstutz, H & LeDuff, M 2006, Background of metal-on-metal resurfacing, *Proc Inst Mech Eng H,* vol. 220, pp. 85-94.

Amstutz, H, Ball, S & LeDuff, M 2007, Early results of conversion of a failed femoral component in hip resurfacing arthroplasty, *J Bone Joint Surg Am,* vol. 89, pp. 735-41.

Antoniou, J, Huk, L, Minarik, W, Mwale, F, Petit ,A & Zukor, D 2008, Metal ion levels in the blood of patients after hip resurfacing: a comparison between twenty-eight and thirty-six-millimeter-head metal-on-metal prostheses, *J Bone Joint Surg Am,* vol. 90, no. 3, pp. 142-8.

Back, D, Bare, J & Shimmin, A 2005, Complications associated with hip resurfacing arthroplasty, *Orthop Clin North Am,* vol. 36, no. 2, pp. 187-93.

Back, D, Dalziel, R, Shimmin, A & Young, D 2005, Early results of primary Birmingham hip resurfacings: an independent prospective study of the first 230 hips, *J Bone Joint Surg Br,* vol. 87, no. 3, pp. 324-9.

Bozic, K, Ludeman, M, Pui, C, Silverstein, M & Vail, T 2010, Do the potential benefits of metal-on-metal hip resurfacing justify the increased cost and risk of complications? *Clin Orthop Relat Res,* vol. 468, pp. 2301-12.

Brazzelli, M, Grant , A, McCormack, K, Vale, L & Wyness, L 2004, The effectiveness of metal-on-metal hip resurfacing: a systematic review of the available evidence published before 2002, *BMC Health Serv Res,* vol. 4, no. 1, pp. 39.

Bruening, W, Chapell, R, Coates, V, Erinoff, E, Kaczmarek, J, Kuserk, E, Schoelles, K & Snyder, D 2006, *Horizon scan on hip replacement surgery,* viewed 15 October 2017, < http://www.cms.gov/Medicare/Coverage/DeterminationProcess/downloads/id44ta.pdf >

California Technology Assessment Forum 2007, *Metal-on-metal total hip resurfacing as an alternative to total hip arthroplasty: a technology assessment,* viewed 15 October 2017, <http://www.etsad.fr/etsad/afficher_lien.php?id=3089>

Cohen, D 2012, How safe are metal-on-metal hip implants? *BMJ,* vol. 344 no. e1410, viewed 15 October 2013, BMJ database, doi: http://dx.doi.org/10.1136/bmj.e1410

Daniel, J, McMinn, D & Pynsent, P 2004, Metal-on-metal resurfacing of the hip in patients under the age of 55 years with osteoarthritis, *J Bone Joint Surg Br,* vol. 86, pp. 177-84.

Dayan, A & Paine, A 2001, Mechanisms of chromium toxicity, carcinogenicity and allergenicity: review of the literature from 1985 to 2000, *Human & Experimental Toxocity,* vol. 20, no. 9, pp. 439-451.

Dettori, J, Ecker, E, Hashimoto, R & Moran, K 2013, *Hip resurfacing update: draft evidence report,* viewed 15 October 2017, < http://www.hta.hca.wa.gov/documents/hip_draft_report_082313.pdf >

Duncan, C, Garbuz, D, Greidanus, N, Masri, B & Tanzer, M 2010, The John Charnley award: metal-on-metal hip resurfacing versus large-diameter head metal-on-metal total hip arthroplasty: a randomized clinical trial, *Clin Orthop Relat Res,* vol. 468, pp. 318-25.

Girard, J, Lavigne, M & Venditolli, A 2006, Biomechanical reconstruction of the hip: a randomized clinical trial comparing total hip resurfacing and total hip arthroplasty. *J Bone Joint Surg,* vol. 88, pp. 721-726.

Karliner, L 2010, *Metal-on-metal hip resurfacing as an alternative to total hip arthroplasty: a technology assessment,* viewed 15 October 2017, <http://www.medscape.com/viewarticle/730321>

Kaulback, K, Levin, L & Sehatzadeh, S 2012, Metal-on-metal hip resurfacing arthroplasty: an analysis of safety and revision rates, *Ont Health Technol Assess Ser,* vol. 12, no. 19, pp. 1-63.

Ladon, D, Doherty, A, Newson, R, Turner, J, Bhamra, M & Case C 2004, Changes in metal levels and chromosome aberrations in the peripheral blood of patients after metal-on-metal hip arthroplasty, *J Arthroplasty,* vol. 19, no. 3, pp. 78-83.

Lee, R, McIsaac, M & Noseworthy, T 2007, *Hip replacement and resurfacing: current considerations regarding metal-on-metal arthroplasty,* viewed 15 October 2017, < http://www.health.alberta.ca/documents/AHTDP-MoMHR-UofC-STE.pdf>

Schrag, D 2013, *Metal-on-metal hip & joint implants FDA-CDRH request for comments - effective date of requirements for pre-market approval for two class III preamendments devices,* viewed 15 October 2017, < http://www.washingtonadvocatesforpatientsafety.org/wp-content/uploads/2013/05/Schrag-FDA-Docket-Comments-4-18-2013.pdf >

YOUR KNOWLEDGE HAS VALUE

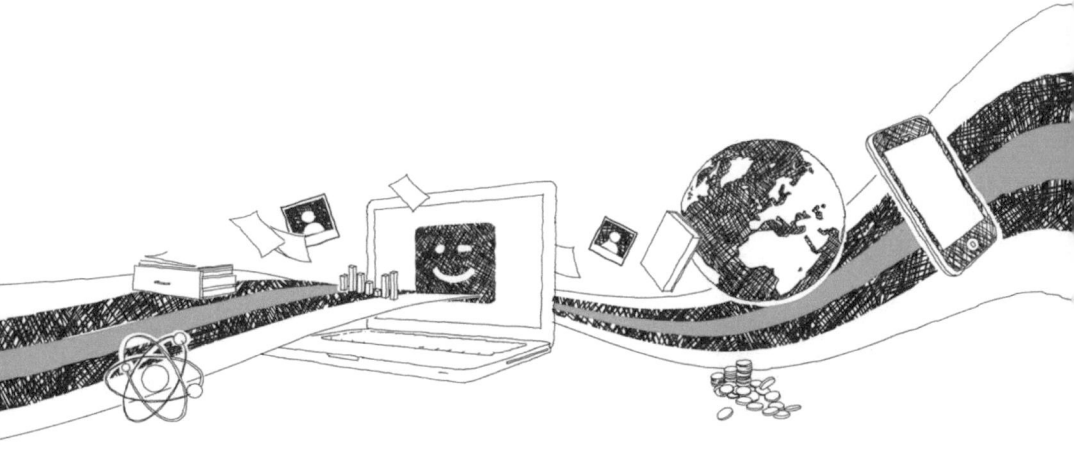

- We will publish your bachelor's and master's thesis, essays and papers

- Your own eBook and book - sold worldwide in all relevant shops

- Earn money with each sale

Upload your text at www.GRIN.com and publish for free

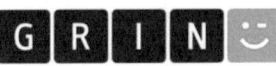